<u>**To use this journal simply fill in the columns:**</u>

- Time
- Type of food and how much/portion size
- Your degree of hunger from 1 -10
- Location

These details will provide insight into emotional triggers for eating habits, as well as times of day and places where healthy and unhealthy foods are most likely to be consumed.

How detailed you are is up to you. I recommend you start with just the bare basics to get in the habit and add details as you continue to log your food over the weeks. However the more thorough you are when recording what you eat (those 5 M&Ms at the office, the extra mayo on your sandwich, the sauce on your dinner) the more ways you'll eventually find to cut those extra calories. When you look back over your food diary records, look for those nibbles and bites that really do add up. Did you know that 150 extra calories in a day (that could be one beer or glass of wine or an extra splash of spread on your sandwich) could result in a 14 to 20 lb weight gain in **one year**?

<u>**On the lined page**</u> write down anything you think is important, such as how you felt (physically and emotionally) when you finished eating, what and how much exercise you got today, any medication you have taken, and your blood sugar results, if you have diabetes.

<u>**Be aware of the common roadblocks many people face.**</u>

*These are the four most common obstacles to keeping a food diary.*

- Are you embarrassed or ashamed about your eating?
- Do you have a sense of hopelessness? Feeling that it won't help to fill out a food diary or that weight loss is impossible for you?
- Does it seem too inconvenient to write down what you eat/drink?
- Do you feel bad when you "slip up"?

<u>**What's the cure?**</u>

- All of these roadblocks can be overcome by remembering the usefulness of the journals
- Not trying to be perfect
- Knowing that slips will happen
- And staying motivated to use tools that promote health and well-being

Date:

| Time | Food & Portion Size | Hunger | Location |
|---|---|---|---|
|  |  |  |  |
|  |  |  |  |
|  |  |  |  |
|  |  |  |  |
|  |  |  |  |
|  |  |  |  |
|  |  |  |  |
|  |  |  |  |

Water ☐ ☐ ☐ ☐ ☐ ☐ ☐ ☐ ☐ ☐ ☐

Date:

| Time | Food & Portion Size | Hunger | Location |
|---|---|---|---|
|  |  |  |  |
|  |  |  |  |
|  |  |  |  |
|  |  |  |  |
|  |  |  |  |
|  |  |  |  |
|  |  |  |  |
|  |  |  |  |
| Water | ☐ ☐ ☐ ☐ ☐ ☐ ☐ ☐ ☐ ☐ ☐ | | |

## Date:

| Time | Food & Portion Size | Hunger | Location |
|------|---------------------|--------|----------|
|      |                     |        |          |
|      |                     |        |          |
|      |                     |        |          |
|      |                     |        |          |
|      |                     |        |          |
|      |                     |        |          |
|      |                     |        |          |
|      |                     |        |          |
| Water | ☐ ☐ ☐ ☐ ☐ ☐ ☐ ☐ ☐ ☐ ☐ | | |

## Date:

| Time | Food & Portion Size | Hunger | Location |
|---|---|---|---|
|  |  |  |  |
|  |  |  |  |
|  |  |  |  |
|  |  |  |  |
|  |  |  |  |
|  |  |  |  |
|  |  |  |  |
|  |  |  |  |
| Water | ☐ ☐ ☐ ☐ ☐ ☐ ☐ ☐ ☐ ☐ ☐ | | |

## Date:

| Time | Food & Portion Size | Hunger | Location |
|------|---------------------|--------|----------|
|      |                     |        |          |
|      |                     |        |          |
|      |                     |        |          |
|      |                     |        |          |
|      |                     |        |          |
|      |                     |        |          |
|      |                     |        |          |
|      |                     |        |          |

Water ☐ ☐ ☐ ☐ ☐ ☐ ☐ ☐ ☐ ☐ ☐

Date:

| Time | Food & Portion Size | Hunger | Location |
|---|---|---|---|
|  |  |  |  |
|  |  |  |  |
|  |  |  |  |
|  |  |  |  |
|  |  |  |  |
|  |  |  |  |
|  |  |  |  |
|  |  |  |  |

Water: ☐ ☐ ☐ ☐ ☐ ☐ ☐ ☐ ☐ ☐ ☐

## Date:

| Time | Food & Portion Size | Hunger | Location |
|------|--------------------|--------|----------|
|      |                    |        |          |
|      |                    |        |          |
|      |                    |        |          |
|      |                    |        |          |
|      |                    |        |          |
|      |                    |        |          |
|      |                    |        |          |
|      |                    |        |          |
| Water | ☐ ☐ ☐ ☐ ☐ ☐ ☐ ☐ ☐ ☐ ☐ | | |

Date:

| Time | Food & Portion Size | Hunger | Location |
|---|---|---|---|
|  |  |  |  |
|  |  |  |  |
|  |  |  |  |
|  |  |  |  |
|  |  |  |  |
|  |  |  |  |
|  |  |  |  |
|  |  |  |  |

| Water | ☐ ☐ ☐ ☐ ☐ ☐ ☐ ☐ ☐ ☐ ☐ |
|---|---|

Date:

| Time | Food & Portion Size | Hunger | Location |
|---|---|---|---|
|  |  |  |  |
|  |  |  |  |
|  |  |  |  |
|  |  |  |  |
|  |  |  |  |
|  |  |  |  |
|  |  |  |  |
|  |  |  |  |

Water ☐ ☐ ☐ ☐ ☐ ☐ ☐ ☐ ☐ ☐ ☐

## Date:

| Time | Food & Portion Size | Hunger | Location |
|---|---|---|---|
|  |  |  |  |
|  |  |  |  |
|  |  |  |  |
|  |  |  |  |
|  |  |  |  |
|  |  |  |  |
|  |  |  |  |
|  |  |  |  |
| Water | ☐ ☐ ☐ ☐ ☐ ☐ ☐ ☐ ☐ ☐ ☐ | | |

## Date:

| Time | Food & Portion Size | Hunger | Location |
|---|---|---|---|
|  |  |  |  |
|  |  |  |  |
|  |  |  |  |
|  |  |  |  |
|  |  |  |  |
|  |  |  |  |
|  |  |  |  |
|  |  |  |  |

Water ☐ ☐ ☐ ☐ ☐ ☐ ☐ ☐ ☐ ☐ ☐

## Date:

| Time | Food & Portion Size | Hunger | Location |
|---|---|---|---|
| | | | |
| | | | |
| | | | |
| | | | |
| | | | |
| | | | |
| | | | |
| | | | |
| Water | ☐ ☐ ☐ ☐ ☐ ☐ ☐ ☐ ☐ ☐ ☐ | | |

Date:

| Time | Food & Portion Size | Hunger | Location |
|------|---------------------|--------|----------|
|      |                     |        |          |
|      |                     |        |          |
|      |                     |        |          |
|      |                     |        |          |
|      |                     |        |          |
|      |                     |        |          |
|      |                     |        |          |
|      |                     |        |          |

Water ☐ ☐ ☐ ☐ ☐ ☐ ☐ ☐ ☐ ☐ ☐

## Date:

| Time | Food & Portion Size | Hunger | Location |
|---|---|---|---|
|  |  |  |  |
|  |  |  |  |
|  |  |  |  |
|  |  |  |  |
|  |  |  |  |
|  |  |  |  |
|  |  |  |  |
|  |  |  |  |

Water ☐ ☐ ☐ ☐ ☐ ☐ ☐ ☐ ☐ ☐ ☐

Date:

| Time | Food & Portion Size | Hunger | Location |
|------|---------------------|--------|----------|
|      |                     |        |          |
|      |                     |        |          |
|      |                     |        |          |
|      |                     |        |          |
|      |                     |        |          |
|      |                     |        |          |
|      |                     |        |          |
|      |                     |        |          |

Water ☐ ☐ ☐ ☐ ☐ ☐ ☐ ☐ ☐ ☐ ☐

Date:

| Time | Food & Portion Size | Hunger | Location |
|---|---|---|---|
|  |  |  |  |
|  |  |  |  |
|  |  |  |  |
|  |  |  |  |
|  |  |  |  |
|  |  |  |  |
|  |  |  |  |
|  |  |  |  |

| Water | ☐ ☐ ☐ ☐ ☐ ☐ ☐ ☐ ☐ ☐ ☐ ☐ |
|---|---|

Date:

| Time | Food & Portion Size | Hunger | Location |
|---|---|---|---|
|  |  |  |  |
|  |  |  |  |
|  |  |  |  |
|  |  |  |  |
|  |  |  |  |
|  |  |  |  |
|  |  |  |  |
|  |  |  |  |

| Water | ☐ ☐ ☐ ☐ ☐ ☐ ☐ ☐ ☐ ☐ ☐ |
|---|---|

Date:

| Time | Food & Portion Size | Hunger | Location |
|---|---|---|---|
|  |  |  |  |
|  |  |  |  |
|  |  |  |  |
|  |  |  |  |
|  |  |  |  |
|  |  |  |  |
|  |  |  |  |
|  |  |  |  |

Water ☐ ☐ ☐ ☐ ☐ ☐ ☐ ☐ ☐ ☐ ☐

Date:

| Time | Food & Portion Size | Hunger | Location |
|---|---|---|---|
|  |  |  |  |
|  |  |  |  |
|  |  |  |  |
|  |  |  |  |
|  |  |  |  |
|  |  |  |  |
|  |  |  |  |
|  |  |  |  |

Water ☐ ☐ ☐ ☐ ☐ ☐ ☐ ☐ ☐ ☐ ☐

## Date:

| Time | Food & Portion Size | Hunger | Location |
|---|---|---|---|
|  |  |  |  |
|  |  |  |  |
|  |  |  |  |
|  |  |  |  |
|  |  |  |  |
|  |  |  |  |
|  |  |  |  |
|  |  |  |  |
| Water | ☐ ☐ ☐ ☐ ☐ ☐ ☐ ☐ ☐ ☐ ☐ | | |

Date:

| Time | Food & Portion Size | Hunger | Location |
|------|---------------------|--------|----------|
|      |                     |        |          |
|      |                     |        |          |
|      |                     |        |          |
|      |                     |        |          |
|      |                     |        |          |
|      |                     |        |          |
|      |                     |        |          |
|      |                     |        |          |
| Water | ☐ ☐ ☐ ☐ ☐ ☐ ☐ ☐ ☐ ☐ ☐ | | |

## Date:

| Time | Food & Portion Size | Hunger | Location |
|---|---|---|---|
|  |  |  |  |
|  |  |  |  |
|  |  |  |  |
|  |  |  |  |
|  |  |  |  |
|  |  |  |  |
|  |  |  |  |
|  |  |  |  |

Water ☐ ☐ ☐ ☐ ☐ ☐ ☐ ☐ ☐ ☐ ☐

Date:

| Time | Food & Portion Size | Hunger | Location |
|---|---|---|---|
|  |  |  |  |
|  |  |  |  |
|  |  |  |  |
|  |  |  |  |
|  |  |  |  |
|  |  |  |  |
|  |  |  |  |
|  |  |  |  |
| Water | ☐ ☐ ☐ ☐ ☐ ☐ ☐ ☐ ☐ ☐ ☐ | | |

Date:

| Time | Food & Portion Size | Hunger | Location |
|------|---------------------|--------|----------|
|      |                     |        |          |
|      |                     |        |          |
|      |                     |        |          |
|      |                     |        |          |
|      |                     |        |          |
|      |                     |        |          |
|      |                     |        |          |
|      |                     |        |          |

Water ☐ ☐ ☐ ☐ ☐ ☐ ☐ ☐ ☐ ☐ ☐

## Date:

| Time | Food & Portion Size | Hunger | Location |
|---|---|---|---|
|  |  |  |  |
|  |  |  |  |
|  |  |  |  |
|  |  |  |  |
|  |  |  |  |
|  |  |  |  |
|  |  |  |  |
|  |  |  |  |
| Water | ☐ ☐ ☐ ☐ ☐ ☐ ☐ ☐ ☐ ☐ ☐ | | |

## Date:

| Time | Food & Portion Size | Hunger | Location |
|---|---|---|---|
|  |  |  |  |
|  |  |  |  |
|  |  |  |  |
|  |  |  |  |
|  |  |  |  |
|  |  |  |  |
|  |  |  |  |
|  |  |  |  |

| Water | ☐ ☐ ☐ ☐ ☐ ☐ ☐ ☐ ☐ ☐ ☐ |
|---|---|

Date:

| Time | Food & Portion Size | Hunger | Location |
|------|---------------------|--------|----------|
|      |                     |        |          |
|      |                     |        |          |
|      |                     |        |          |
|      |                     |        |          |
|      |                     |        |          |
|      |                     |        |          |
|      |                     |        |          |
|      |                     |        |          |

Water ☐ ☐ ☐ ☐ ☐ ☐ ☐ ☐ ☐ ☐ ☐

## Date:

| Time | Food & Portion Size | Hunger | Location |
|------|---------------------|--------|----------|
|      |                     |        |          |
|      |                     |        |          |
|      |                     |        |          |
|      |                     |        |          |
|      |                     |        |          |
|      |                     |        |          |
|      |                     |        |          |
|      |                     |        |          |
| Water | ☐ ☐ ☐ ☐ ☐ ☐ ☐ ☐ ☐ ☐ ☐ | | |

Date:

| Time | Food & Portion Size | Hunger | Location |
|---|---|---|---|
|  |  |  |  |
|  |  |  |  |
|  |  |  |  |
|  |  |  |  |
|  |  |  |  |
|  |  |  |  |
|  |  |  |  |
|  |  |  |  |

Water ☐ ☐ ☐ ☐ ☐ ☐ ☐ ☐ ☐ ☐ ☐

Date:

| Time | Food & Portion Size | Hunger | Location |
|---|---|---|---|
|  |  |  |  |
|  |  |  |  |
|  |  |  |  |
|  |  |  |  |
|  |  |  |  |
|  |  |  |  |
|  |  |  |  |
|  |  |  |  |

Water □ □ □ □ □ □ □ □ □ □ □

## Date:

| Time | Food & Portion Size | Hunger | Location |
|------|---------------------|--------|----------|
|      |                     |        |          |
|      |                     |        |          |
|      |                     |        |          |
|      |                     |        |          |
|      |                     |        |          |
|      |                     |        |          |
|      |                     |        |          |
|      |                     |        |          |

| Water | ☐ ☐ ☐ ☐ ☐ ☐ ☐ ☐ ☐ ☐ |
|-------|---------------------|

## Date:

| Time | Food & Portion Size | Hunger | Location |
|------|---------------------|--------|----------|
|      |                     |        |          |
|      |                     |        |          |
|      |                     |        |          |
|      |                     |        |          |
|      |                     |        |          |
|      |                     |        |          |
|      |                     |        |          |
|      |                     |        |          |

Water ☐ ☐ ☐ ☐ ☐ ☐ ☐ ☐ ☐ ☐ ☐

Date:

| Time | Food & Portion Size | Hunger | Location |
| --- | --- | --- | --- |
|  |  |  |  |
|  |  |  |  |
|  |  |  |  |
|  |  |  |  |
|  |  |  |  |
|  |  |  |  |
|  |  |  |  |
|  |  |  |  |

Water ☐ ☐ ☐ ☐ ☐ ☐ ☐ ☐ ☐ ☐ ☐

Date:

| Time | Food & Portion Size | Hunger | Location |
|------|---------------------|--------|----------|
|      |                     |        |          |
|      |                     |        |          |
|      |                     |        |          |
|      |                     |        |          |
|      |                     |        |          |
|      |                     |        |          |
|      |                     |        |          |
|      |                     |        |          |

Water ☐ ☐ ☐ ☐ ☐ ☐ ☐ ☐ ☐ ☐ ☐

## Date:

| Time | Food & Portion Size | Hunger | Location |
|------|---------------------|--------|----------|
|      |                     |        |          |
|      |                     |        |          |
|      |                     |        |          |
|      |                     |        |          |
|      |                     |        |          |
|      |                     |        |          |
|      |                     |        |          |
|      |                     |        |          |

Water ☐ ☐ ☐ ☐ ☐ ☐ ☐ ☐ ☐ ☐ ☐

Date:

| Time | Food & Portion Size | Hunger | Location |
|------|---------------------|--------|----------|
|      |                     |        |          |
|      |                     |        |          |
|      |                     |        |          |
|      |                     |        |          |
|      |                     |        |          |
|      |                     |        |          |
|      |                     |        |          |
|      |                     |        |          |
| Water | ☐ ☐ ☐ ☐ ☐ ☐ ☐ ☐ ☐ ☐ ☐ | | |

## Date:

| Time | Food & Portion Size | Hunger | Location |
|------|---------------------|--------|----------|
|  |  |  |  |
|  |  |  |  |
|  |  |  |  |
|  |  |  |  |
|  |  |  |  |
|  |  |  |  |
|  |  |  |  |
|  |  |  |  |

Water  □ □ □ □ □ □ □ □ □ □ □

## Date:

| Time | Food & Portion Size | Hunger | Location |
|------|---------------------|--------|----------|
|      |                     |        |          |
|      |                     |        |          |
|      |                     |        |          |
|      |                     |        |          |
|      |                     |        |          |
|      |                     |        |          |
|      |                     |        |          |
|      |                     |        |          |

Water ☐ ☐ ☐ ☐ ☐ ☐ ☐ ☐ ☐ ☐ ☐

## Date:

| Time | Food & Portion Size | Hunger | Location |
|------|---------------------|--------|----------|
|      |                     |        |          |
|      |                     |        |          |
|      |                     |        |          |
|      |                     |        |          |
|      |                     |        |          |
|      |                     |        |          |
|      |                     |        |          |
|      |                     |        |          |

Water ☐ ☐ ☐ ☐ ☐ ☐ ☐ ☐ ☐ ☐ ☐

Date:

| Time | Food & Portion Size | Hunger | Location |
|------|---------------------|--------|----------|
|      |                     |        |          |
|      |                     |        |          |
|      |                     |        |          |
|      |                     |        |          |
|      |                     |        |          |
|      |                     |        |          |
|      |                     |        |          |
|      |                     |        |          |
| Water | ☐ ☐ ☐ ☐ ☐ ☐ ☐ ☐ ☐ ☐ ☐ | | |

Date:

| Time | Food & Portion Size | Hunger | Location |
|---|---|---|---|
|  |  |  |  |
|  |  |  |  |
|  |  |  |  |
|  |  |  |  |
|  |  |  |  |
|  |  |  |  |
|  |  |  |  |
|  |  |  |  |

Water ☐ ☐ ☐ ☐ ☐ ☐ ☐ ☐ ☐ ☐ ☐

Date:

| Time | Food & Portion Size | Hunger | Location |
|------|---------------------|--------|----------|
|      |                     |        |          |
|      |                     |        |          |
|      |                     |        |          |
|      |                     |        |          |
|      |                     |        |          |
|      |                     |        |          |
|      |                     |        |          |
|      |                     |        |          |

Water ☐ ☐ ☐ ☐ ☐ ☐ ☐ ☐ ☐ ☐ ☐

Date:

| Time | Food & Portion Size | Hunger | Location |
| --- | --- | --- | --- |
|  |  |  |  |
|  |  |  |  |
|  |  |  |  |
|  |  |  |  |
|  |  |  |  |
|  |  |  |  |
|  |  |  |  |
|  |  |  |  |

Water ☐ ☐ ☐ ☐ ☐ ☐ ☐ ☐ ☐ ☐ ☐

## Date:

| Time | Food & Portion Size | Hunger | Location |
|------|---------------------|--------|----------|
|      |                     |        |          |
|      |                     |        |          |
|      |                     |        |          |
|      |                     |        |          |
|      |                     |        |          |
|      |                     |        |          |
|      |                     |        |          |
|      |                     |        |          |
| Water | ☐ ☐ ☐ ☐ ☐ ☐ ☐ ☐ ☐ ☐ ☐ | | |

## Date:

| Time | Food & Portion Size | Hunger | Location |
|------|---------------------|--------|----------|
|      |                     |        |          |
|      |                     |        |          |
|      |                     |        |          |
|      |                     |        |          |
|      |                     |        |          |
|      |                     |        |          |
|      |                     |        |          |
|      |                     |        |          |

| Water | ☐ ☐ ☐ ☐ ☐ ☐ ☐ ☐ ☐ ☐ ☐ |
|-------|-------------------------|

Date:

| Time | Food & Portion Size | Hunger | Location |
|------|---------------------|--------|----------|
|      |                     |        |          |
|      |                     |        |          |
|      |                     |        |          |
|      |                     |        |          |
|      |                     |        |          |
|      |                     |        |          |
|      |                     |        |          |
|      |                     |        |          |

Water ☐ ☐ ☐ ☐ ☐ ☐ ☐ ☐ ☐ ☐ ☐

## Date:

| Time | Food & Portion Size | Hunger | Location |
|---|---|---|---|
|  |  |  |  |
|  |  |  |  |
|  |  |  |  |
|  |  |  |  |
|  |  |  |  |
|  |  |  |  |
|  |  |  |  |
|  |  |  |  |

Water ☐ ☐ ☐ ☐ ☐ ☐ ☐ ☐ ☐ ☐ ☐

## Date:

| Time | Food & Portion Size | Hunger | Location |
|------|---------------------|--------|----------|
|      |                     |        |          |
|      |                     |        |          |
|      |                     |        |          |
|      |                     |        |          |
|      |                     |        |          |
|      |                     |        |          |
|      |                     |        |          |
|      |                     |        |          |

| Water | ☐ ☐ ☐ ☐ ☐ ☐ ☐ ☐ ☐ ☐ ☐ |
|-------|------------------------|

Date:

| Time | Food & Portion Size | Hunger | Location |
|---|---|---|---|
|  |  |  |  |
|  |  |  |  |
|  |  |  |  |
|  |  |  |  |
|  |  |  |  |
|  |  |  |  |
|  |  |  |  |
|  |  |  |  |

Water ☐ ☐ ☐ ☐ ☐ ☐ ☐ ☐ ☐ ☐ ☐

Date:

| Time | Food & Portion Size | Hunger | Location |
|------|---------------------|--------|----------|
|      |                     |        |          |
|      |                     |        |          |
|      |                     |        |          |
|      |                     |        |          |
|      |                     |        |          |
|      |                     |        |          |
|      |                     |        |          |
|      |                     |        |          |

Water ☐ ☐ ☐ ☐ ☐ ☐ ☐ ☐ ☐ ☐ ☐

## Date:

| Time | Food & Portion Size | Hunger | Location |
|------|---------------------|--------|----------|
|      |                     |        |          |
|      |                     |        |          |
|      |                     |        |          |
|      |                     |        |          |
|      |                     |        |          |
|      |                     |        |          |
|      |                     |        |          |
|      |                     |        |          |

**Water** ☐ ☐ ☐ ☐ ☐ ☐ ☐ ☐ ☐ ☐

Date:

| Time | Food & Portion Size | Hunger | Location |
|------|---------------------|--------|----------|
|      |                     |        |          |
|      |                     |        |          |
|      |                     |        |          |
|      |                     |        |          |
|      |                     |        |          |
|      |                     |        |          |
|      |                     |        |          |
|      |                     |        |          |
| Water | ☐ ☐ ☐ ☐ ☐ ☐ ☐ ☐ ☐ ☐ ☐ | | |

Date:

| Time | Food & Portion Size | Hunger | Location |
|---|---|---|---|
|  |  |  |  |
|  |  |  |  |
|  |  |  |  |
|  |  |  |  |
|  |  |  |  |
|  |  |  |  |
|  |  |  |  |
|  |  |  |  |
| Water | ☐ ☐ ☐ ☐ ☐ ☐ ☐ ☐ ☐ ☐ ☐ | | |

Date:

| Time | Food & Portion Size | Hunger | Location |
|------|---------------------|--------|----------|
|      |                     |        |          |
|      |                     |        |          |
|      |                     |        |          |
|      |                     |        |          |
|      |                     |        |          |
|      |                     |        |          |
|      |                     |        |          |
|      |                     |        |          |
| Water | ☐ ☐ ☐ ☐ ☐ ☐ ☐ ☐ ☐ ☐ ☐ | | |

Date:

| Time | Food & Portion Size | Hunger | Location |
|---|---|---|---|
|  |  |  |  |
|  |  |  |  |
|  |  |  |  |
|  |  |  |  |
|  |  |  |  |
|  |  |  |  |
|  |  |  |  |
|  |  |  |  |

Water   ☐ ☐ ☐ ☐ ☐ ☐ ☐ ☐ ☐ ☐ ☐

Date:

| Time | Food & Portion Size | Hunger | Location |
|---|---|---|---|
| | | | |
| | | | |
| | | | |
| | | | |
| | | | |
| | | | |
| | | | |
| | | | |

Water ☐ ☐ ☐ ☐ ☐ ☐ ☐ ☐ ☐ ☐ ☐

## Date:

| Time | Food & Portion Size | Hunger | Location |
|---|---|---|---|
|  |  |  |  |
|  |  |  |  |
|  |  |  |  |
|  |  |  |  |
|  |  |  |  |
|  |  |  |  |
|  |  |  |  |
|  |  |  |  |
| Water | ☐ ☐ ☐ ☐ ☐ ☐ ☐ ☐ ☐ ☐ | | |

## Date:

| Time | Food & Portion Size | Hunger | Location |
|---|---|---|---|
|  |  |  |  |
|  |  |  |  |
|  |  |  |  |
|  |  |  |  |
|  |  |  |  |
|  |  |  |  |
|  |  |  |  |
|  |  |  |  |
| Water | ☐ ☐ ☐ ☐ ☐ ☐ ☐ ☐ ☐ ☐ ☐ | | |

Date:

| Time | Food & Portion Size | Hunger | Location |
|---|---|---|---|
| | | | |
| | | | |
| | | | |
| | | | |
| | | | |
| | | | |
| | | | |
| | | | |
| Water | ☐ ☐ ☐ ☐ ☐ ☐ ☐ ☐ ☐ ☐ | | |

## Date:

| Time | Food & Portion Size | Hunger | Location |
|------|--------------------|--------|----------|
|      |                    |        |          |
|      |                    |        |          |
|      |                    |        |          |
|      |                    |        |          |
|      |                    |        |          |
|      |                    |        |          |
|      |                    |        |          |
|      |                    |        |          |
| Water | ☐ ☐ ☐ ☐ ☐ ☐ ☐ ☐ ☐ ☐ ☐ | | |

Date:

| Time | Food & Portion Size | Hunger | Location |
|---|---|---|---|
|  |  |  |  |
|  |  |  |  |
|  |  |  |  |
|  |  |  |  |
|  |  |  |  |
|  |  |  |  |
|  |  |  |  |
|  |  |  |  |

Water □ □ □ □ □ □ □ □ □ □ □

Date:

| Time | Food & Portion Size | Hunger | Location |
|---|---|---|---|
|  |  |  |  |
|  |  |  |  |
|  |  |  |  |
|  |  |  |  |
|  |  |  |  |
|  |  |  |  |
|  |  |  |  |
|  |  |  |  |
| Water | ☐ ☐ ☐ ☐ ☐ ☐ ☐ ☐ ☐ ☐ ☐ | | |

## Date:

| Time | Food & Portion Size | Hunger | Location |
|---|---|---|---|
|  |  |  |  |
|  |  |  |  |
|  |  |  |  |
|  |  |  |  |
|  |  |  |  |
|  |  |  |  |
|  |  |  |  |
|  |  |  |  |

Water ☐ ☐ ☐ ☐ ☐ ☐ ☐ ☐ ☐ ☐ ☐

Date:

| Time | Food & Portion Size | Hunger | Location |
|------|---------------------|--------|----------|
|      |                     |        |          |
|      |                     |        |          |
|      |                     |        |          |
|      |                     |        |          |
|      |                     |        |          |
|      |                     |        |          |
|      |                     |        |          |
|      |                     |        |          |

Water ☐ ☐ ☐ ☐ ☐ ☐ ☐ ☐ ☐ ☐ ☐

Date:

| Time | Food & Portion Size | Hunger | Location |
|---|---|---|---|
|  |  |  |  |
|  |  |  |  |
|  |  |  |  |
|  |  |  |  |
|  |  |  |  |
|  |  |  |  |
|  |  |  |  |
|  |  |  |  |

Water ☐ ☐ ☐ ☐ ☐ ☐ ☐ ☐ ☐ ☐ ☐

## Date:

| Time | Food & Portion Size | Hunger | Location |
|---|---|---|---|
| | | | |
| | | | |
| | | | |
| | | | |
| | | | |
| | | | |
| | | | |
| | | | |

**Water** ☐ ☐ ☐ ☐ ☐ ☐ ☐ ☐ ☐ ☐ ☐

## Date:

| Time | Food & Portion Size | Hunger | Location |
|------|---------------------|--------|----------|
|      |                     |        |          |
|      |                     |        |          |
|      |                     |        |          |
|      |                     |        |          |
|      |                     |        |          |
|      |                     |        |          |
|      |                     |        |          |
|      |                     |        |          |

Water ☐ ☐ ☐ ☐ ☐ ☐ ☐ ☐ ☐ ☐ ☐

Date:

| Time | Food & Portion Size | Hunger | Location |
| --- | --- | --- | --- |
|  |  |  |  |
|  |  |  |  |
|  |  |  |  |
|  |  |  |  |
|  |  |  |  |
|  |  |  |  |
|  |  |  |  |
|  |  |  |  |
| Water | ☐ ☐ ☐ ☐ ☐ ☐ ☐ ☐ ☐ ☐ ☐ | | |

Date:

| Time | Food & Portion Size | Hunger | Location |
| --- | --- | --- | --- |
|  |  |  |  |
|  |  |  |  |
|  |  |  |  |
|  |  |  |  |
|  |  |  |  |
|  |  |  |  |
|  |  |  |  |
|  |  |  |  |

Water ☐ ☐ ☐ ☐ ☐ ☐ ☐ ☐ ☐ ☐ ☐

Date:

| Time | Food & Portion Size | Hunger | Location |
|---|---|---|---|
|  |  |  |  |
|  |  |  |  |
|  |  |  |  |
|  |  |  |  |
|  |  |  |  |
|  |  |  |  |
|  |  |  |  |
|  |  |  |  |

Water ☐ ☐ ☐ ☐ ☐ ☐ ☐ ☐ ☐ ☐ ☐

## Date:

| Time | Food & Portion Size | Hunger | Location |
|------|---------------------|--------|----------|
|      |                     |        |          |
|      |                     |        |          |
|      |                     |        |          |
|      |                     |        |          |
|      |                     |        |          |
|      |                     |        |          |
|      |                     |        |          |
|      |                     |        |          |

| Water | ☐ ☐ ☐ ☐ ☐ ☐ ☐ ☐ ☐ ☐ ☐ |
|-------|------------------------|

Date:

| Time | Food & Portion Size | Hunger | Location |
|------|---------------------|--------|----------|
|      |                     |        |          |
|      |                     |        |          |
|      |                     |        |          |
|      |                     |        |          |
|      |                     |        |          |
|      |                     |        |          |
|      |                     |        |          |
|      |                     |        |          |
| Water | ☐ ☐ ☐ ☐ ☐ ☐ ☐ ☐ ☐ ☐ ☐ | | |

Date:

| Time | Food & Portion Size | Hunger | Location |
| --- | --- | --- | --- |
|  |  |  |  |
|  |  |  |  |
|  |  |  |  |
|  |  |  |  |
|  |  |  |  |
|  |  |  |  |
|  |  |  |  |
|  |  |  |  |
| Water | ☐ ☐ ☐ ☐ ☐ ☐ ☐ ☐ ☐ ☐ ☐ | | |

Date:

| Time | Food & Portion Size | Hunger | Location |
|------|---------------------|--------|----------|
|      |                     |        |          |
|      |                     |        |          |
|      |                     |        |          |
|      |                     |        |          |
|      |                     |        |          |
|      |                     |        |          |
|      |                     |        |          |
|      |                     |        |          |

Water ☐ ☐ ☐ ☐ ☐ ☐ ☐ ☐ ☐ ☐ ☐

Date:

| Time | Food & Portion Size | Hunger | Location |
|------|---------------------|--------|----------|
|      |                     |        |          |
|      |                     |        |          |
|      |                     |        |          |
|      |                     |        |          |
|      |                     |        |          |
|      |                     |        |          |
|      |                     |        |          |
|      |                     |        |          |

Water ☐ ☐ ☐ ☐ ☐ ☐ ☐ ☐ ☐ ☐ ☐

## Date:

| Time | Food & Portion Size | Hunger | Location |
|------|---------------------|--------|----------|
|      |                     |        |          |
|      |                     |        |          |
|      |                     |        |          |
|      |                     |        |          |
|      |                     |        |          |
|      |                     |        |          |
|      |                     |        |          |
|      |                     |        |          |

| Water | ☐ ☐ ☐ ☐ ☐ ☐ ☐ ☐ ☐ ☐ ☐ |
|-------|------------------------|

Date:

| Time | Food & Portion Size | Hunger | Location |
|---|---|---|---|
|  |  |  |  |
|  |  |  |  |
|  |  |  |  |
|  |  |  |  |
|  |  |  |  |
|  |  |  |  |
|  |  |  |  |
|  |  |  |  |

Water ☐ ☐ ☐ ☐ ☐ ☐ ☐ ☐ ☐ ☐ ☐

## Date:

| Time | Food & Portion Size | Hunger | Location |
|---|---|---|---|
|  |  |  |  |
|  |  |  |  |
|  |  |  |  |
|  |  |  |  |
|  |  |  |  |
|  |  |  |  |
|  |  |  |  |
|  |  |  |  |

Water ☐ ☐ ☐ ☐ ☐ ☐ ☐ ☐ ☐ ☐ ☐

Date:

| Time | Food & Portion Size | Hunger | Location |
|---|---|---|---|
|  |  |  |  |
|  |  |  |  |
|  |  |  |  |
|  |  |  |  |
|  |  |  |  |
|  |  |  |  |
|  |  |  |  |
|  |  |  |  |

Water ☐ ☐ ☐ ☐ ☐ ☐ ☐ ☐ ☐ ☐ ☐

Date:

| Time | Food & Portion Size | Hunger | Location |
|------|---------------------|--------|----------|
|      |                     |        |          |
|      |                     |        |          |
|      |                     |        |          |
|      |                     |        |          |
|      |                     |        |          |
|      |                     |        |          |
|      |                     |        |          |
|      |                     |        |          |

Water ☐ ☐ ☐ ☐ ☐ ☐ ☐ ☐ ☐ ☐ ☐

Date:

| Time | Food & Portion Size | Hunger | Location |
|------|---------------------|--------|----------|
|      |                     |        |          |
|      |                     |        |          |
|      |                     |        |          |
|      |                     |        |          |
|      |                     |        |          |
|      |                     |        |          |
|      |                     |        |          |
|      |                     |        |          |

| Water | ☐ ☐ ☐ ☐ ☐ ☐ ☐ ☐ ☐ ☐ ☐ |
|-------|------------------------|

Date:

| Time | Food & Portion Size | Hunger | Location |
|------|---------------------|--------|----------|
|      |                     |        |          |
|      |                     |        |          |
|      |                     |        |          |
|      |                     |        |          |
|      |                     |        |          |
|      |                     |        |          |
|      |                     |        |          |
|      |                     |        |          |

Water ☐ ☐ ☐ ☐ ☐ ☐ ☐ ☐ ☐ ☐ ☐

## Date:

| Time | Food & Portion Size | Hunger | Location |
|---|---|---|---|
|  |  |  |  |
|  |  |  |  |
|  |  |  |  |
|  |  |  |  |
|  |  |  |  |
|  |  |  |  |
|  |  |  |  |
|  |  |  |  |

| Water | ☐ ☐ ☐ ☐ ☐ ☐ ☐ ☐ ☐ ☐ |
|---|---|

## Date:

| Time | Food & Portion Size | Hunger | Location |
|------|---------------------|--------|----------|
|      |                     |        |          |
|      |                     |        |          |
|      |                     |        |          |
|      |                     |        |          |
|      |                     |        |          |
|      |                     |        |          |
|      |                     |        |          |
|      |                     |        |          |

| Water | ☐ ☐ ☐ ☐ ☐ ☐ ☐ ☐ ☐ ☐ ☐ |
|-------|------------------------|

Date:

| Time | Food & Portion Size | Hunger | Location |
|---|---|---|---|
|  |  |  |  |
|  |  |  |  |
|  |  |  |  |
|  |  |  |  |
|  |  |  |  |
|  |  |  |  |
|  |  |  |  |
|  |  |  |  |
| Water | ☐ ☐ ☐ ☐ ☐ ☐ ☐ ☐ ☐ ☐ ☐ | | |

## Date:

| Time | Food & Portion Size | Hunger | Location |
|------|---------------------|--------|----------|
|      |                     |        |          |
|      |                     |        |          |
|      |                     |        |          |
|      |                     |        |          |
|      |                     |        |          |
|      |                     |        |          |
|      |                     |        |          |
|      |                     |        |          |

| Water | ☐ ☐ ☐ ☐ ☐ ☐ ☐ ☐ ☐ ☐ ☐ |
|-------|------------------------|

## Date:

| Time | Food & Portion Size | Hunger | Location |
|---|---|---|---|
|  |  |  |  |
|  |  |  |  |
|  |  |  |  |
|  |  |  |  |
|  |  |  |  |
|  |  |  |  |
|  |  |  |  |
|  |  |  |  |

| Water | ☐ ☐ ☐ ☐ ☐ ☐ ☐ ☐ ☐ ☐ ☐ |
|---|---|

Date:

| Time | Food & Portion Size | Hunger | Location |
|------|---------------------|--------|----------|
|      |                     |        |          |
|      |                     |        |          |
|      |                     |        |          |
|      |                     |        |          |
|      |                     |        |          |
|      |                     |        |          |
|      |                     |        |          |
|      |                     |        |          |
| Water | ☐ ☐ ☐ ☐ ☐ ☐ ☐ ☐ ☐ ☐ ☐ | | |

Date:

| Time | Food & Portion Size | Hunger | Location |
| --- | --- | --- | --- |
|  |  |  |  |
|  |  |  |  |
|  |  |  |  |
|  |  |  |  |
|  |  |  |  |
|  |  |  |  |
|  |  |  |  |
|  |  |  |  |
| Water | ☐ ☐ ☐ ☐ ☐ ☐ ☐ ☐ ☐ ☐ ☐ | | |

Date:

| Time | Food & Portion Size | Hunger | Location |
|---|---|---|---|
|  |  |  |  |
|  |  |  |  |
|  |  |  |  |
|  |  |  |  |
|  |  |  |  |
|  |  |  |  |
|  |  |  |  |
|  |  |  |  |

Water ☐ ☐ ☐ ☐ ☐ ☐ ☐ ☐ ☐ ☐ ☐

## Date:

| Time | Food & Portion Size | Hunger | Location |
|------|---------------------|--------|----------|
|      |                     |        |          |
|      |                     |        |          |
|      |                     |        |          |
|      |                     |        |          |
|      |                     |        |          |
|      |                     |        |          |
|      |                     |        |          |
|      |                     |        |          |
| Water | ☐ ☐ ☐ ☐ ☐ ☐ ☐ ☐ ☐ ☐ ☐ | | |

## Date:

| Time | Food & Portion Size | Hunger | Location |
|---|---|---|---|
|  |  |  |  |
|  |  |  |  |
|  |  |  |  |
|  |  |  |  |
|  |  |  |  |
|  |  |  |  |
|  |  |  |  |
|  |  |  |  |

Water ☐ ☐ ☐ ☐ ☐ ☐ ☐ ☐ ☐ ☐ ☐

## Date:

| Time | Food & Portion Size | Hunger | Location |
|---|---|---|---|
| | | | |
| | | | |
| | | | |
| | | | |
| | | | |
| | | | |
| | | | |
| | | | |

| Water | ☐ ☐ ☐ ☐ ☐ ☐ ☐ ☐ ☐ ☐ ☐ |
|---|---|

Date:

| Time | Food & Portion Size | Hunger | Location |
|---|---|---|---|
|  |  |  |  |
|  |  |  |  |
|  |  |  |  |
|  |  |  |  |
|  |  |  |  |
|  |  |  |  |
|  |  |  |  |
|  |  |  |  |
| Water | ☐ ☐ ☐ ☐ ☐ ☐ ☐ ☐ ☐ ☐ ☐ | | |

Date:

| Time | Food & Portion Size | Hunger | Location |
| --- | --- | --- | --- |
|  |  |  |  |
|  |  |  |  |
|  |  |  |  |
|  |  |  |  |
|  |  |  |  |
|  |  |  |  |
|  |  |  |  |
|  |  |  |  |

Water ☐ ☐ ☐ ☐ ☐ ☐ ☐ ☐ ☐ ☐ ☐

## Date:

| Time | Food & Portion Size | Hunger | Location |
|---|---|---|---|
|  |  |  |  |
|  |  |  |  |
|  |  |  |  |
|  |  |  |  |
|  |  |  |  |
|  |  |  |  |
|  |  |  |  |
|  |  |  |  |

Water ☐ ☐ ☐ ☐ ☐ ☐ ☐ ☐ ☐ ☐ ☐

## Date:

| Time | Food & Portion Size | Hunger | Location |
|------|---------------------|--------|----------|
|      |                     |        |          |
|      |                     |        |          |
|      |                     |        |          |
|      |                     |        |          |
|      |                     |        |          |
|      |                     |        |          |
|      |                     |        |          |
|      |                     |        |          |
| Water | ☐ ☐ ☐ ☐ ☐ ☐ ☐ ☐ ☐ ☐ ☐ | | |

## Date:

| Time | Food & Portion Size | Hunger | Location |
|------|---------------------|--------|----------|
|      |                     |        |          |
|      |                     |        |          |
|      |                     |        |          |
|      |                     |        |          |
|      |                     |        |          |
|      |                     |        |          |
|      |                     |        |          |
|      |                     |        |          |

Water ☐ ☐ ☐ ☐ ☐ ☐ ☐ ☐ ☐ ☐ ☐

## Date:

| Time | Food & Portion Size | Hunger | Location |
|---|---|---|---|
|  |  |  |  |
|  |  |  |  |
|  |  |  |  |
|  |  |  |  |
|  |  |  |  |
|  |  |  |  |
|  |  |  |  |
|  |  |  |  |

Water ☐ ☐ ☐ ☐ ☐ ☐ ☐ ☐ ☐ ☐ ☐

AMAZING!

You made it to the end of this journal!

Now take a few minutes to look back and see how far you have come and celebrate that **_you did it!_**

Congratulations on all your success and sticking with it but this isn't the end of the journey. Keep logging your food every day to ensure you keep those pounds from creeping back!

-- Trish Vroom